MTHFR DIET COOKBOOK

Essential Meal Plans and Recipes for

Optimal

Health and Genetic Support

BY

HELEN HOLLIS

Table of contents

INTRODUCTION

Welcome to the MTHFR Diet Cookbook

Essential Meal Plans and Recipes for Optimal Health and Genetic Support." Whether you're newly diagnosed with an MTHFR mutation or looking to optimize your health through diet, you've taken a crucial step towards better well-being by picking up this book.

This cookbook is more than just a collection of recipes; it's a comprehensive guide designed to support your genetic health through carefully crafted meal plans and delicious dishes.

Each recipe is tailored to enhance your body's ability to manage the challenges posed by MTHFR mutations, helping you to thrive and feel your best.

Understanding MTHFR

Before we dive into the culinary delights, it's important to understand the foundation of the MTHFR diet. MTHFR stands for methylenetetrahydrofolate reductase, an enzyme that plays a key role in processing amino acids, the building blocks of proteins. Specifically, MTHFR is crucial in converting folate (vitamin B9) into its active form, which your body needs to perform a myriad of essential functions.

However, certain genetic mutations can impair the function of this enzyme, leading to a variety of health issues ranging from fatigue and brain fog to more serious conditions like cardiovascular diseases and pregnancy complications. By adopting a diet that supports MTHFR function, you can mitigate these risks and enhance your overall health.

The Importance of Diet in Managing MTHFR

Diet plays a pivotal role in managing MTHFR mutations.

A well-balanced diet rich in specific nutrients can significantly improve your body's methylation processes and overall health.

This cookbook focuses on nutrient-dense foods that support detoxification, reduce inflammation, and boost your energy levels.

Key components of the MTHFR diet include

Folate-Rich Foods: Natural sources of folate like leafy greens, legumes, and certain fruits.

Vitamin B12 and B6: These vitamins are essential for proper methylation and can be found in meats, fish, and dairy.

Antioxidant-Rich Foods: Fruits, vegetables, nuts, and seeds that combat oxidative stress.

Gluten-Free and Low-Processed Foods: To reduce inflammation and support gut health.

How to Use This Cookbook

This cookbook is designed to be your companion in the kitchen, offering a variety of recipes that cater to different tastes and dietary needs while keeping your genetic health in mind. Here's how to make the most of it:

Start with the Basics: The initial chapters provide foundational knowledge about the MTHFR mutation and essential nutrients. Take the time to understand these sections to fully grasp the importance of the recipes that follow.

Plan Your Meals: Use the meal planning tips and grocery shopping guide to organize your weekly menus.

This will save you time and ensure you're always prepared with healthy, MTHFR-friendly options.

Explore the Recipes: Dive into the diverse array of recipes, from hearty breakfasts to satisfying dinners, snacks, and desserts. Each recipe includes detailed instructions and nutritional information to help you make informed choices.

Follow the Meal Plans: The 4-week meal plan for beginners is a great way to kickstart your journey. Follow it closely to experience the benefits of the MTHFR diet firsthand.

Customize to Your Needs: Everyone's genetic makeup and health needs are unique. Feel free to adjust the recipes and meal plans to suit your preferences and dietary requirements.

CHAPTER ONE: Getting Started with the MTHFR Diet

Essential Nutrients for MTHFR

Managing MTHFR mutations effectively begins with understanding the essential nutrients that support optimal methylation and overall health. Incorporating these nutrients into your daily diet can make a significant difference in how you feel and function.

Folate (Vitamin B9): Folate is critical for DNA synthesis and repair, as well as for converting homocysteine to methionine, a process vital for detoxification and overall health.

Choose natural sources like leafy greens (spinach, kale), legumes (lentils, beans), avocados, and citrus fruits.

Vitamin B12: This vitamin is essential for nerve function, red blood cell formation, and DNA synthesis. It works intimately with folate in the methylation cycle. Foods rich in B12 include meat, fish, dairy products, and fortified plant-based milks.

Vitamin B6: Vitamin B6 is involved in over 100 enzyme reactions in the body, most of which are concerned with protein metabolism. It's found in food varieties like poultry, fish, potatoes, chickpeas, and bananas.

Riboflavin (Vitamin B2): Riboflavin helps convert food into energy and supports cellular function, growth, and development. Sources include eggs, lean meats, green vegetables, and almonds.

Magnesium: Magnesium is vital for hundreds of biochemical reactions in the body, including energy production and DNA synthesis. It's found in nuts, seeds, whole grains, and green leafy vegetables.

Cancer prevention agent: Cell reinforcements assist with shielding your cells from harm brought about by free revolutionaries. Incorporate a variety of colorful fruits and vegetables, nuts, and seeds to ensure a good intake of antioxidants.

Foods to Include and Avoid

Knowing which foods to include and which to avoid can help you manage your MTHFR mutation more effectively.

Foods to Include:

Leafy Greens: Spinach, kale, Swiss chard, and arugula are excellent sources of folate. Cruciferous Vegetables: Broccoli, Brussels sprouts, cauliflower, and cabbage support detoxification.

Whole Grains: Quinoa, earthy colored rice, and oats give fundamental supplements and fiber. Lean Proteins: Chicken, turkey, fish, eggs, and legumes offer B vitamins and protein.

Nuts and Seeds: Almonds, pecans, chia seeds, and flax seeds are wealthy in magnesium and solid fats.

Berries and Fruits: Blueberries, strawberries, oranges, and avocados are packed with antioxidants and vitamins. Healthy Fats: Olive oil, coconut oil, and fatty fish like salmon provide anti-inflammatory benefits.

Foods to Avoid:

Processed Foods: These often contain unhealthy fats, sugars, and additives that can exacerbate inflammation.
Gluten-Containing Grains: Wheat, barley, and rye can trigger sensitivities in some people with MTHFR mutations.

Refined Sugars and Artificial Sweeteners: These can disrupt metabolic processes and increase oxidative stress.
Alcohol: Excessive consumption can interfere with methylation and deplete essential nutrients.

Meal Planning Tips and Tricks

Effective meal planning is key to maintaining a balanced diet that supports your MTHFR mutation.

Here are a few hints and deceives to assist you with getting everything rolling:

Prepare: Take a period every week to design your feasts. This can assist you with settling on better decisions and stay away from somewhat late, less nutritious choices.

Clump Cooking: Plan enormous amounts of specific feasts and freeze segments for some other time. This is particularly valuable for occupied days.

Diverse Ingredients: Ensure your meal plans include a variety of foods to cover all essential nutrients. Rotate recipes to keep things interesting.

Portion Control: Be aware of piece sizes to try not to indulge. Use smaller plates if necessary to help with this.

Hydration: Drink plenty of water throughout the day to support overall health and detoxification.

Grocery Shopping Guide

Navigating the grocery store can be daunting, but with a well-prepared list, you can make healthier choices with ease. Here's a guide to help you shop for your MTHFR diet:

Produce Section: Spend most of your time here. Stock up on leafy greens, colorful vegetables, and fresh fruits.

Meat and Fish: Choose lean proteins like chicken, turkey, and fatty fish such as salmon and mackerel.

Dairy and Alternatives: Look for organic or grass-fed options. Consider fortified plant-based milks if you're avoiding dairy.

Grains and Legumes: Opt for whole grains like quinoa, brown rice, and gluten-free oats. Include a variety of beans and lentils.

Nuts and Seeds: Almonds, walnuts, chia seeds, and flaxseeds are great to have on hand for snacks and meal additions.

Oils and Fats: Select high-quality oils such as extra virgin olive oil, coconut oil, and avocado oil.

Herbs and Spices: Fresh and dried herbs and spices add flavor and additional nutrients to your meals.

Frozen Section: Frozen fruits and vegetables are a convenient and nutritious option, especially when certain produce is out of season.

By focusing on these essential nutrients, foods, and tips, you'll be well-equipped to manage your MTHFR mutation through diet.

CHAPTER TWO:
BREAKFAST RECIPES

Superfood Smoothie Bow

Description: Kickstart your day with this nutrient-dense smoothie bowl packed with antioxidants, vitamins, and minerals. It's a vibrant and refreshing way to get your daily dose of fruits and leafy greens.

Prep Time: 10 minutes
Cook Time: 0 minutes
Serving: 1 bowl

Nutritional Information: Calories: 250, Protein: 6g, Carbohydrates: 45g, Fat: 6g, Fiber: 8g

Ingredients:

- 1 cup fresh spinach
- 1/2 cup frozen mixed berries
- 1/2 banana
- 1/2 cup almond milk (unsweetened)
- 1 tablespoon chia seeds
- 1 tablespoon almond butter
- 1 teaspoon honey (optional)

Toppings: sliced banana, fresh berries, granola, shredded coconut

Preparation Instructions:

- In a blender, combine spinach, frozen berries, banana, almond milk, chia seeds, almond butter, and honey.
- Blend until smooth and creamy. Adjust the consistency by adding more almond milk if necessary.
- Pour the smoothie into a bowl and top with sliced banana, fresh berries, granola, and shredded coconut.
- Enjoy immediately with a spoon.

Gluten-Free Almond Pancakes

Description: Light and fluffy, these gluten-free almond pancakes are a perfect breakfast treat. They are rich in protein and healthy fats, making them a satisfying start to your day.

Prep Time: 10 minutes
Cook Time: 15 minutes
Serving: 4 pancakes

Nutritional Information: Calories: 200, Protein: 8g, Carbohydrates: 12g, Fat: 14g, Fiber: 3g

Ingredients:

- 1 cup almond flour
- 2 eggs
- 1/4 cup unsweetened almond milk
- 1 tablespoon honey
- 1/2 teaspoon baking powder
- 1/4 teaspoon salt
- 1 teaspoon vanilla extract
- Coconut oil for cooking

Preparation Instructions:

- In a medium bowl, whisk together almond flour, eggs, almond milk, honey, baking powder, salt, and vanilla extract until smooth.
- Heat a non-stick skillet over medium heat and lightly grease with coconut oil.

- Pour 1/4 cup of batter onto the skillet for each pancake. Cook until bubbles form on the surface, about 2-3 minutes.
- Flip the pancakes and cook for another 2-3 minutes until golden brown.
- Serve warm with your favorite toppings such as fresh berries, almond butter, or a drizzle of maple syrup.

Quinoa Breakfast Porridge

Description: This hearty quinoa breakfast porridge is a nutritious alternative to traditional oatmeal. Packed with protein and fiber, it's a great way to keep you full and energized throughout the morning.

Prep Time: 5 minutes
Cook Time: 20 minutes
Serving: 2 servings

Nutritional Information: Calories: 300, Protein: 10g, Carbohydrates: 50g, Fat: 8g, Fiber: 6g

Ingredients:

- 1 cup cooked quinoa
- 1 cup unsweetened almond milk
- 1 tablespoon chia seeds
- 1 tablespoon maple syrup
- 1 teaspoon cinnamon
- 1/2 teaspoon vanilla extract

Toppings: sliced banana, fresh berries, chopped nuts

Preparation Instructions:

- In a medium saucepan, combine cooked quinoa, almond milk, chia seeds, maple syrup, cinnamon, and vanilla extract.
- Bring to a simmer over medium heat, stirring occasionally.

- Cook for 10-15 minutes until the porridge thickens to your desired consistency.
- Divide the porridge into bowls and top with sliced banana, fresh berries, and chopped nuts.
- Serve warm and enjoy.

Egg Muffins with Spinach and Feta

Description: These savory egg muffins are perfect for meal prepping. They are packed with protein and greens, making them a convenient and healthy breakfast option.

Prep Time: 10 minutes
Cook Time: 20 minutes
Serving: 6 muffins

Nutritional Information: Calories: 100, Protein: 8g, Carbohydrates: 2g, Fat: 7g, Fiber: 1g

Ingredients:

- 6 large eggs
- 1/2 cup fresh spinach, chopped
- 1/4 cup crumbled feta cheese
- 1/4 cup diced red bell pepper
- 1/4 cup diced onion
- Salt and pepper to taste
- Coconut oil for greasing

Preparation Instructions:

- Preheat the oven to 375°F (190°C). Grease a muffin tin with coconut oil.
- In a large bowl, whisk the eggs until well beaten.
- Add chopped spinach, feta cheese, bell pepper, onion, salt, and pepper to the eggs. Stir to combine.

- Pour the egg mixture evenly into the muffin tin.
- Bake for 20 minutes, or until the egg muffins are set and slightly golden.
- Allow to cool for a few minutes before removing from the tin.
- Store in the refrigerator for up to 5 days. Reheat in the microwave before serving.

Avocado Toast with a Twist

Description: Avocado toast is a classic breakfast favorite, and this version adds a twist with a variety of toppings to boost its nutritional value and flavor.

Prep Time: 10 minutes
Cook Time: 0 minutes
Serving: 2 servings

Nutritional Information: Calories: 250, Protein: 6g, Carbohydrates: 28g, Fat: 14g, Fiber: 8g

Ingredients:

- 2 slices of gluten-free bread
- 1 ripe avocado
- 1 tablespoon lemon juice
- Salt and pepper to taste

Toppings: sliced cherry tomatoes, radishes, microgreens, hemp seeds

Preparation Instructions:

- Toast the gluten-free bread slices until golden brown.
- In a small bowl, mash the avocado with lemon juice, salt, and pepper.
- Spread the mashed avocado evenly onto the toasted bread slices.

- Top with sliced cherry tomatoes, radishes, microgreens, and a sprinkle of hemp seeds.
- Serve immediately and enjoy.

These breakfast recipes are designed to provide a nutritious start to your day, supporting your health and well-being as you manage your MTHFR mutation. Enjoy exploring these delicious options!

Kale And Quinoa Salad

Description: This vibrant and nutritious salad combines the earthy flavors of kale with the nutty taste of quinoa, creating a satisfying meal rich in protein, fiber, and antioxidants.

Prep Time: 15 minutes
Cook Time: 15 minutes
Serving: 4 servings

Nutritional Information: Calories: 250, Protein: 8g, Carbohydrates: 30g, Fat: 10g, Fiber: 5g

Ingredients:

-
  - 1 cup quinoa, rinsed
  - 2 cups water
  - 4 cups kale, chopped
  - 1/2 cup cherry tomatoes, halved
  - 1/4 cup red onion, thinly sliced
  - 1/4 cup crumbled feta cheese
  - 1/4 cup chopped almonds
  - 1/4 cup dried cranberries

Dressing:

- 1/4 cup olive oil
- 2 tablespoons lemon juice
- 1 tablespoon honey
- 1 teaspoon Dijon mustard
- Salt and pepper to taste

Preparation Instructions:

- In a medium saucepan, bring the quinoa and water to a boil.
- Reduce the heat to low, cover, and simmer for 15 minutes or until the quinoa is tender and the water is absorbed.
- Fluff with a fork and let cool.
- In a large bowl, combine the chopped kale, cherry tomatoes, red onion, feta

cheese, almonds, and dried cranberries.

- In a small bowl, whisk together the olive oil, lemon juice, honey, Dijon mustard, salt, and pepper.
- Add the cooled quinoa to the kale mixture and drizzle with the dressing. Toss to combine.
- Serve immediately or refrigerate until ready to eat.

Chicken And Avocado Wraps

Description: These delicious and easy-to-make wraps are filled with tender chicken, creamy avocado, and crisp vegetables, making them a perfect lunch option for a quick and healthy meal.

Prep Time: 15 minutes
Cook Time: 10 minutes
Serving: 4 wraps

Nutritional Information: Calories: 350, Protein: 25g, Carbohydrates: 30g, Fat: 15g, Fiber: 8g

Ingredients:

- 2 cooked chicken breasts, shredded
- 1 avocado, sliced
- 1 cup mixed greens
- 1/2 cup cherry tomatoes, halved
- 1/4 cup red onion, thinly sliced
- 4 whole wheat or gluten-free tortillas
- 1/4 cup hummus
- 1 tablespoon lime juice
- Salt and pepper to taste

Preparation Instructions:

- In a medium bowl, combine the shredded chicken, lime juice, salt, and pepper.
- Lay the tortillas flat and spread each with a thin layer of hummus.

- Arrange the mixed greens, cherry tomatoes, red onion, avocado slices, and chicken mixture evenly on each tortilla.
- Roll up the tortillas tightly and slice in half.
- Serve immediately or wrap in foil for a convenient lunch on the go.

Lentil And Vegetable Soup

Description: This hearty lentil and vegetable soup is packed with plant-based protein, fiber, and a variety of colorful vegetables, making it a comforting and nutritious lunch option.

Prep Time: 15 minutes
Cook Time: 30 minutes
Serving: 6 servings

Nutritional Information: Calories: 200, Protein: 10g, Carbohydrates: 35g, Fat: 4g, Fiber: 12g

Ingredients:

- 1 cup green or brown lentils, rinsed
- 1 tablespoon olive oil
- 1 onion, diced
- 2 garlic cloves, minced
- 2 carrots, diced
- 2 celery stalks, diced
- 1 zucchini, diced
- 1 red bell pepper, diced
- 1 can (14.5 oz) diced tomatoes
- 6 cups vegetable broth
- 1 teaspoon dried thyme
- 1 teaspoon dried basil
- Salt and pepper to taste
- 2 cups fresh spinach, chopped

Preparation Instructions:

- In a large pot, heat the olive oil over medium heat. Add the onion and garlic and sauté until softened, about 5 minutes.
- Add the carrots, celery, zucchini, and red bell pepper. Cook for another 5 minutes.
- Stir in the lentils, diced tomatoes, vegetable broth, thyme, basil, salt, and pepper.
- Bring the soup to a boil, then reduce the heat and simmer for 25-30 minutes, or until the lentils and vegetables are tender.
- Stir in the fresh spinach and cook for an additional 2-3 minutes, until wilted.

- Serve hot with a side of whole-grain bread if desired.

Mediterranean Chickpea Salad

Description: This refreshing Mediterranean chickpea salad is bursting with flavors from fresh vegetables, herbs, and a tangy lemon dressing. It's a light yet satisfying lunch option.

Prep Time: 15 minutes

Cook Time: 0 minutes

Serving: 4 servings

Nutritional Information: Calories: 300, Protein: 10g, Carbohydrates: 40g, Fat: 12g, Fiber: 10g

Ingredients:

- 2 cans (15 oz each) chickpeas, rinsed and drained
- 1 cup cherry tomatoes, halved
- 1 cucumber, diced
- 1/4 cup red onion, finely chopped
- 1/4 cup Kalamata olives, pitted and sliced
- 1/4 cup crumbled feta cheese
- 1/4 cup fresh parsley, chopped

Dressing:

- 1/4 cup olive oil
- 2 tablespoons lemon juice
- 1 teaspoon dried oregano
- Salt and pepper to taste

Preparation Instructions:

- In a large bowl, combine the chickpeas, cherry tomatoes, cucumber, red onion, olives, feta cheese, and parsley.
- In a small bowl, whisk together the olive oil, lemon juice, oregano, salt, and pepper.
- Pour the dressing over the salad and toss to combine.

- Serve immediately or refrigerate until ready to eat.

Stuffed Bell Peppers

Description: These colorful bell peppers are stuffed with a flavorful mixture of quinoa, black beans, and vegetables, making them a nutritious and filling lunch option.

Prep Time: 15 minutes
Cook Time: 30 minutes
Serving: 4 servings

Nutritional Information: Calories: 300, Protein: 12g, Carbohydrates: 45g, Fat: 8g, Fiber: 12g

Ingredients:

- 4 bell peppers, tops cut off and seeds removed
- 1 cup cooked quinoa
- 1 can (15 oz) black beans, rinsed and drained
- 1/2 cup corn kernels
- 1/2 cup diced tomatoes
- 1/4 cup chopped green onions
- 1/4 cup chopped cilantro
- 1 teaspoon cumin
- 1 teaspoon chili powder
- Salt and pepper to taste
- 1/2 cup shredded cheese (optional)

Preparation Instructions:

- Preheat the oven to 375°F (190°C).
- In a large bowl, combine the cooked quinoa, black beans, corn, diced tomatoes, green onions, cilantro, cumin, chili powder, salt, and pepper.
- Stuff each bell pepper with the quinoa mixture and place them in a baking dish.
- If using, sprinkle shredded cheese on top of each stuffed pepper.
- Cover the dish with foil and bake for 25 minutes. Remove the foil and bake for an additional 5 minutes, until the peppers are tender and the cheese is melted.
- Serve hot and enjoy.

These lunch recipes are designed to provide a variety of flavors and nutrients, ensuring you stay satisfied and energized throughout your day while managing your MTHFR mutation. Enjoy these delicious and wholesome options!

Baked Salmon with Garlic and Dill

Description: This simple yet flavorful baked salmon is enhanced with the fresh flavors of garlic and dill, making it a nutritious and delicious dinner option that's rich in omega-3 fatty acids.

Prep Time: 10 minutes
Cook Time: 20 minutes
Serving: 4 servings

Nutritional Information: Calories: 300, Protein: 25g, Carbohydrates: 2g, Fat: 20g, Fiber: 0g

Ingredients:

- 4 salmon filets
- 3 cloves garlic, minced
- 2 tablespoons fresh dill, chopped
- 2 tablespoons olive oil
- 1 lemon, thinly sliced
- Salt and pepper to taste

Preparation Instructions:

- Preheat the oven to 375°F (190°C).
- Place the salmon filets on a baking sheet lined with parchment paper.

- In a small bowl, mix the minced garlic, chopped dill, olive oil, salt, and pepper.
- Spread the garlic and dill mixture evenly over the salmon filets.
- Top each filet with a few slices of lemon.
- Bake for 18-20 minutes, or until the salmon is cooked through and flakes easily with a fork.
- Serve immediately with your favorite side dishes.

Quinoa-Stuffed Bell Peppers

Description: These colorful bell peppers are stuffed with a savory mixture of quinoa, black beans, and vegetables, making them a nutritious and satisfying dinner option.

Prep Time: 15 minutes
Cook Time: 30 minutes
Serving: 4 servings

Nutritional Information: Calories: 350, Protein: 12g, Carbohydrates: 50g, Fat: 10g, Fiber: 10g

Ingredients:

- 4 bell peppers, tops cut off and seeds removed
- 1 cup cooked quinoa
- 1 can (15 oz) black beans, rinsed and drained
- 1/2 cup corn kernels
- 1/2 cup diced tomatoes
- 1/4 cup chopped green onions
- 1/4 cup chopped cilantro
- 1 teaspoon cumin
- 1 teaspoon chili powder
- Salt and pepper to taste
- 1/2 cup shredded cheese (optional)

Preparation Instructions:

- Preheat the oven to 375°F (190°C).
- In a large bowl, combine the cooked quinoa, black beans, corn, diced tomatoes, green onions, cilantro, cumin, chili powder, salt, and pepper.
- Stuff each bell pepper with the quinoa mixture and place them in a baking dish.
- If using, sprinkle shredded cheese on top of each stuffed pepper.
- Cover the dish with foil and bake for 25 minutes. Remove the foil and bake for an additional 5 minutes, until the peppers are tender and the cheese is melted.
- Serve hot and enjoy.

Lemon Herb Chicken Skewers

Description: These juicy chicken skewers are marinated in a lemon herb dressing, then grilled to perfection. They're a tasty and healthy option for a quick and easy dinner.

Prep Time: 15 minutes (plus 30 minutes to marinate)
Cook Time: 15 minutes
Serving: 4 servings

Nutritional Information: Calories: 250, Protein: 30g, Carbohydrates: 4g, Fat: 12g, Fiber: 1g

Ingredients:

- 4 boneless, skinless chicken breasts, cut into 1-inch pieces
- 3 tablespoons olive oil
- 2 tablespoons lemon juice
- 2 cloves garlic, minced
- 1 tablespoon fresh rosemary, chopped
- 1 tablespoon fresh thyme, chopped
- 1 teaspoon salt
- 1/2 teaspoon black pepper
- Wooden skewers, soaked in water

Preparation Instructions:

- In a large bowl, mix the olive oil, lemon juice, garlic, rosemary, thyme, salt, and pepper.
- Add the chicken pieces to the bowl and toss to coat. Cover and marinate in the refrigerator for at least 30 minutes.
- Preheat the grill to medium-high heat.
- Thread the marinated chicken pieces onto the soaked skewers.
- Grill the skewers for 12-15 minutes, turning occasionally, until the chicken is cooked through and has a nice char.
- Serve immediately with a side salad or grilled vegetables.

Zucchini Noodles with Pesto

Description: This light and flavorful dish features zucchini noodles tossed with a fresh basil pesto. It's a low-carb, nutrient-rich dinner that's perfect for a quick and healthy meal.

Prep Time: 15 minutes
Cook Time: 5 minutes
Serving: 4 servings

Nutritional Information: Calories: 200, Protein: 6g, Carbohydrates: 10g, Fat: 16g, Fiber: 4g

Ingredients:

- 4 medium zucchinis, spiralized into noodles
- 1 cup fresh basil leaves
- 1/4 cup pine nuts
- 1/4 cup grated Parmesan cheese
- 2 cloves garlic
- 1/4 cup olive oil
- Salt and pepper to taste

Preparation Instructions:

- In a food processor, combine the basil leaves, pine nuts, Parmesan cheese, and garlic. Pulse until finely chopped.
- With the processor running, slowly add the olive oil until the pesto is

smooth. Season with salt and pepper to taste.

- In a large skillet, heat a small amount of olive oil over medium heat. Add the zucchini noodles and sauté for 2-3 minutes, until just tender.

- Remove from heat and toss the zucchini noodles with the pesto until well coated.

- Serve immediately, garnished with extra Parmesan cheese and pine nuts if desired.

Turkey Meatballs with Marinara Sauce

Description: These tender turkey meatballs are cooked in a rich marinara sauce, making them a comforting and healthy dinner option that's perfect for the whole family.

Prep Time: 20 minutes
Cook Time: 30 minutes
Serving: 4 servings

Nutritional Information: Calories: 350, Protein: 25g, Carbohydrates: 20g, Fat: 18g, Fiber: 4g

Ingredients:

- 1 pound ground turkey
- 1/4 cup almond flour
- 1/4 cup grated Parmesan cheese
- 1 egg
- 2 cloves garlic, minced
- 1 tablespoon fresh parsley, chopped
- 1 teaspoon dried oregano
- Salt and pepper to taste
- 2 cups marinara sauce
- 1 tablespoon olive oil

Preparation Instructions:

- In a large bowl, combine the ground turkey, almond flour, Parmesan cheese, egg, garlic, parsley, oregano, salt, and pepper. Mix until well combined.

- Form the mixture into small meatballs, about 1 inch in diameter.
- In a large skillet, heat the olive oil over medium heat. Add the meatballs and cook until browned on all sides, about 5-7 minutes.
- Pour the marinara sauce over the meatballs, reduce the heat to low, and simmer for 20-25 minutes, until the meatballs are cooked through.
- Serve hot with spaghetti squash or zucchini noodles for a low-carb option.

Eggplant Parmesan

Description: This lighter version of the classic Italian dish features breaded and baked eggplant slices layered with marinara sauce and cheese, creating a delicious and satisfying dinner.

Prep Time: 20 minutes
Cook Time: 40 minutes
Serving: 4 servings

Nutritional Information: Calories: 400, Protein: 15g, Carbohydrates: 45g, Fat: 20g, Fiber: 10g

Ingredients:

- 2 large eggplants, sliced into 1/4-inch rounds
- 1 cup almond flour
- 2 eggs, beaten
- 2 cups marinara sauce
- 1 1/2 cups shredded mozzarella cheese
- 1/2 cup grated Parmesan cheese
- 1 tablespoon dried Italian seasoning
- Salt and pepper to taste
- Olive oil spray

Preparation Instructions:

- Preheat the oven to 375°F (190°C). Line a baking sheet with parchment paper.

- Dip each eggplant slice in the beaten eggs, then coat with almond flour. Place the slices on the prepared baking sheet.

- Lightly spray the eggplant slices with olive oil. Bake for 20 minutes, flipping halfway through, until golden and crispy.

- In a large baking dish, spread a thin layer of marinara sauce. Arrange a layer of eggplant slices over the sauce.

- Sprinkle it with mozzarella cheese and Parmesan cheese. Repeat the layers, ending with a layer of cheese on top.

- Bake for 20-25 minutes, until the cheese is melted and bubbly.

- Serve hot, garnished with fresh basil if desired.

CHAPTER THREE: SNACK AND APPETIZER RECIPES

Spicy Roasted Chickpeas

Description: These crispy roasted chickpeas are seasoned with a blend of spices for a crunchy, satisfying snack that's packed with protein and fiber.

Prep Time: 10 minutes
Cook Time: 30 minutes
Serving: 4 servings

Nutritional Information: Calories: 180, Protein: 8g, Carbohydrates: 27g, Fat: 6g, Fiber: 6g

Ingredients:

- 1 can (15 oz) chickpeas, rinsed and drained
- 1 tablespoon olive oil
- 1 teaspoon smoked paprika
- 1/2 teaspoon cumin
- 1/2 teaspoon chili powder
- 1/4 teaspoon cayenne pepper (optional)
- Salt to taste

Preparation Instructions:

- Preheat the oven to 400°F (200°C). Line a baking sheet with parchment paper.
- Pat the chickpeas dry with a paper towel and place them in a bowl.
- Toss the chickpeas with olive oil, smoked paprika, cumin, chili powder, cayenne pepper (if using), and salt.
- Spread the chickpeas in a single layer on the prepared baking sheet.
- Roast for 25-30 minutes, shaking the pan halfway through, until the chickpeas are crispy and golden.
- Allow to cool before serving. Store in an airtight container for up to a week.

Veggie-Stuffed Hummus Dip

Description: This colorful and creamy hummus dip is loaded with fresh vegetables, making it a nutritious and delicious appetizer for any occasion.

Prep Time: 15 minutes
Cook Time: 0 minutes
Serving: 6 servings

Nutritional Information: Calories: 150, Protein: 5g, Carbohydrates: 15g, Fat: 8g, Fiber: 4g

Ingredients:

- 1 cup hummus
- 1/2 cup cherry tomatoes, halved
- 1/2 cup diced cucumber
- 1/4 cup diced red bell pepper
- 1/4 cup sliced black olives
- 1/4 cup crumbled feta cheese (optional)
- Fresh parsley for garnish

Preparation Instructions:

- Spread the hummus evenly on a serving platter or dish.
- Top with cherry tomatoes, cucumber, red bell pepper, black olives, and crumbled feta cheese (if using).
- Garnish with fresh parsley.

- Serve with pita chips or fresh vegetable sticks for dipping.

Guacamole with Veggie Chips

Description: This classic guacamole is rich and creamy, perfect for pairing with homemade veggie chips for a wholesome and tasty snack.

Prep Time: 10 minutes
Cook Time: 0 minutes
Serving: 4 servings

Nutritional Information: Calories: 200, Protein: 3g, Carbohydrates: 20g, Fat: 14g, Fiber: 6g

Ingredients:

- 2 ripe avocados
- 1 small onion, finely chopped
- 1 small tomato, diced
- 1 jalapeño, seeded and minced
- 2 tablespoons lime juice
- Salt to taste
- Homemade veggie chips (for serving)

Preparation Instructions:

- In a bowl, mash the avocados with a fork.

- Add the onion, tomato, jalapeño, lime juice, and salt. Mix until well combined.
- Taste and adjust seasoning as needed.
- Serve immediately with homemade veggie chips.

Homemade Veggie Chips:

Prep Time: 10 minutes
Cook Time: 25 minutes
Serving: 4 servings

Nutritional Information: Calories: 150, Protein: 3g, Carbohydrates: 20g, Fat: 7g, Fiber: 4g

Ingredients:

- 2 large sweet potatoes, thinly sliced
- 1 tablespoon olive oil
- 1/2 teaspoon paprika
- 1/2 teaspoon garlic powder
- Salt to taste

Preparation Instructions:

- Preheat the oven to 400°F (200°C). Line a baking sheet with parchment paper.
- Toss the sweet potato slices with olive oil, paprika, garlic powder, and salt.
- Arrange the slices in a single layer on the baking sheet.

- Bake for 20-25 minutes, flipping halfway through, until crisp and golden.
- Cool before serving.

Stuffed Mini Peppers

Description: These bite-sized mini peppers are stuffed with a creamy, herbed cheese filling, making them a delightful and nutritious appetizer.

Prep Time: 15 minutes
Cook Time: 0 minutes
Serving: 4 servings

Nutritional Information: Calories: 120, Protein: 5g, Carbohydrates: 8g, Fat: 8g, Fiber: 2g

Ingredients:

- 12 mini bell peppers, halved and seeded
- 1/2 cup cream cheese, softened
- 1/4 cup Greek yogurt
- 1/4 cup chopped fresh herbs (such as chives, parsley, and dill)
- 1 clove garlic, minced
- Salt and pepper to taste

Preparation Instructions:

- In a bowl, mix the cream cheese, Greek yogurt, fresh herbs, garlic, salt, and pepper until smooth.
- Spoon the mixture into the halved mini bell peppers.
- Arrange on a serving platter.
- Serve immediately or refrigerate until ready to serve.

Almond-Crusted Cheese Bites

Description: These crunchy almond-crusted cheese bites are a great low-carb snack that combines the richness of cheese with the nutty crunch of almonds.

Prep Time: 10 minutes
Cook Time: 15 minutes
Serving: 4 servings

Nutritional Information: Calories: 180, Protein: 10g, Carbohydrates: 4g, Fat: 14g, Fiber: 2g

Ingredients:

- 1 cup shredded cheddar cheese
- 1/2 cup almond flour
- 1/4 cup grated Parmesan cheese
- 1/2 teaspoon paprika
- 1 egg, beaten
- Olive oil spray

Preparation Instructions:

- Preheat the oven to 375°F (190°C). Line a baking sheet with parchment paper.
- In a bowl, mix the shredded cheddar cheese, almond flour, Parmesan cheese, and paprika.

- Roll small portions of the cheese mixture into balls and dip them into the beaten egg.
- warm or at room temperature.

These snack and appetizer recipes are designed to offer a variety of tasty, nutritious options that can support your health while managing your MTHFR mutation. Enjoy these delightful and wholesome snacks!

GREEN POWER SMOOTHIE

Description: This vibrant smoothie combines nutrient-dense greens with refreshing fruit for a boost of vitamins and minerals. It's a great way to start your day or to recharge during a busy afternoon.

Prep Time: 5 minutes
Cook Time: 0 minutes
Serving: 2 servings

Nutritional Information: Calories: 180, Protein: 4g, Carbohydrates: 30g, Fat: 4g, Fiber: 6g

Ingredients:

- 1 cup spinach
- 1 cup kale, stems removed
- 1 banana, peeled
- 1/2 cup frozen mango chunks
- 1/2 cup almond milk
- 1 tablespoon chia seeds
- Juice of 1/2 lemon

Preparation Instructions:

- Place all ingredients into a blender.
- Blend on high until smooth and creamy.

- Pour into glasses and serve immediately.

Berry Blast Smoothie

Description: This delicious smoothie is packed with antioxidant-rich berries and a touch of honey for natural sweetness. It's perfect for a quick breakfast or a healthy snack.

Prep Time: 5 minutes
Cook Time: 0 minutes
Serving: 2 servings

Nutritional Information: Calories: 190, Protein: 5g, Carbohydrates: 35g, Fat: 2g, Fiber: 8g

Ingredients:

- 1/2 cup strawberries, hulled
- 1/2 cup blueberries
- 1/2 cup raspberries
- 1/2 cup Greek yogurt
- 1 tablespoon honey
- 1/2 cup water or almond milk

Preparation Instructions:

- Combine all ingredients in a blender.
- Blend until smooth.
- Pour into glasses and serve immediately.

Tropical Delight Smoothie

Description: This smoothie offers a tropical escape with its blend of pineapple, coconut, and banana. It's both refreshing and satisfying, making it a great choice for a light and energizing drink.

Prep Time: 5 minutes
Cook Time: 0 minutes
Serving: 2 servings

Nutritional Information: Calories: 210, Protein: 3g, Carbohydrates: 45g, Fat: 4g, Fiber: 5g

Ingredients:

- 1 cup pineapple chunks (fresh or frozen)
- 1/2 cup coconut milk
- 1 banana, peeled
- 1 tablespoon flax seeds
- 1/2 cup ice

Preparation Instructions:

- Place all ingredients into a blender.
- Blend on high until smooth and creamy.
- Pour into glasses and serve immediately.

Chocolate Avocado Smoothie

Description: This creamy smoothie combines the rich flavors of chocolate with the creamy texture of avocado. It's a decadent yet healthy treat that's perfect for any time of day.

Prep Time: 5 minutes
Cook Time: 0 minutes
Serving: 2 servings

Nutritional Information: Calories: 250, Protein: 5g, Carbohydrates: 30g, Fat: 15g, Fiber: 7g

Ingredients:

- 1 ripe avocado, peeled and pitted
- 2 tablespoons cocoa powder
- 1/4 cup honey or maple syrup
- 1 cup almond milk
- 1/2 cup ice

Preparation Instructions:

- Combine all ingredients in a blender.
- Blend until smooth.
- Pour into glasses and serve immediately.

Citrus Ginger Detox Drink

Description: This refreshing detox drink combines zesty citrus flavors with the invigorating kick of ginger. It's perfect for cleansing and revitalizing your body.

Prep Time: 10 minutes
Cook Time: 0 minutes
Serving: 2 servings

Nutritional Information: Calories: 60, Protein: 1g, Carbohydrates: 15g, Fat: 0g, Fiber: 2g

Ingredients:

- 1 cup orange juice
- 1/2 cup lemon juice
- 1 tablespoon freshly grated ginger
- 1 tablespoon honey or agave syrup (optional)
- 1 cup cold water

Preparation Instructions:

- In a pitcher, combine the orange juice, lemon juice, grated ginger, and honey (if using).
- Add the cold water and stir well.
- Serve over ice and enjoy.

Creamy Almond Smoothie

Description: This creamy almond smoothie is made with almond butter and a touch of vanilla, offering a deliciously smooth and nutty drink that's perfect for a nutritious snack or breakfast.

Prep Time: 5 minutes
Cook Time: 0 minutes
Serving: 2 servings

Nutritional Information: Calories: 220, Protein: 6g, Carbohydrates: 20g, Fat: 14g, Fiber: 5g

Ingredients:

- 2 tablespoons almond butter
- 1 banana, peeled
- 1 cup almond milk
- 1/2 teaspoon vanilla extract
- 1 tablespoon honey or maple syrup (optional)
- 1/2 cup ice

Preparation Instructions:

- Place all ingredients in a blender.
- Blend until smooth and creamy.
- Pour into glasses and serve immediately.

These smoothie and drink recipes are crafted to be delicious and nourishing, offering a variety of flavors and nutrients to support your health. Enjoy these refreshing options!

Almond Flour Chocolate Chip Cookies

Description: These soft and chewy cookies are made with almond flour and dark chocolate chips, offering a gluten-free and lower-carb alternative to traditional cookies.

Prep Time: 10 minutes
Cook Time: 15 minutes
Serving: 12 cookies

Nutritional Information: Calories: 150, Protein: 4g, Carbohydrates: 15g, Fat: 10g, Fiber: 2g

Ingredients:

- 1 1/2 cups almond flour
- 1/4 cup coconut flour
- 1/2 teaspoon baking soda
- 1/4 teaspoon salt
- 1/4 cup coconut oil, melted
- 1/4 cup honey or maple syrup
- 1 large egg
- 1 teaspoon vanilla extract
- 1/2 cup dark chocolate chips

Preparation Instructions:

- Preheat the oven to 350°F (175°C). Line a baking sheet with parchment paper.
- In a bowl, mix together almond flour, coconut flour, baking soda, and salt.
- In another bowl, combine melted coconut oil, honey, egg, and vanilla extract.
- Stir the wet ingredients into the dry ingredients until well combined.
- Fold in the dark chocolate chips.
- Drop spoonfuls of dough onto the prepared baking sheet.
- Bake for 12-15 minutes, until the edges are golden.

- Allow to cool on the baking sheet for a few minutes before transferring to a wire rack to cool completely.

Berry Chia Seed Pudding

Description: This creamy chia seed pudding is infused with fresh berries and a touch of vanilla, making it a nutritious and delicious dessert that's also rich in fiber.

Prep Time: 10 minutes
Cook Time: 0 minutes
Serving: 4 servings

Nutritional Information: Calories: 180, Protein: 6g, Carbohydrates: 20g, Fat: 8g, Fiber: 10g

Ingredients:

- 1/4 cup chia seeds
- 1 cup almond milk
- 1 tablespoon maple syrup
- 1/2 teaspoon vanilla extract
- 1/2 cup mixed berries (fresh or frozen)

Preparation Instructions:

- In a bowl, whisk together chia seeds, almond milk, maple syrup, and vanilla extract.
- Cover and refrigerate for at least 4 hours or overnight, until thickened.

- Stir well before serving and top with mixed berries.

Coconut Macaroons

Description: These sweet and chewy coconut macaroons are perfect for a quick and satisfying dessert. They're naturally gluten-free and can be enjoyed as a treat or a snack.

Prep Time: 15 minutes
Cook Time: 20 minutes
Serving: 20 macaroons

Nutritional Information: Calories: 110, Protein: 2g, Carbohydrates: 12g, Fat: 7g, Fiber: 2g

Ingredients:

- 2 cups unsweetened shredded coconut
- 1/2 cup egg whites (about 3 large eggs)
- 1/2 cup honey or maple syrup
- 1 teaspoon vanilla extract
- A pinch of salt

Preparation Instructions:

- Preheat the oven to 325°F (165°C). Line a baking sheet with parchment paper.
- In a bowl, mix shredded coconut, egg whites, honey, vanilla extract, and salt.

- Drop tablespoon-sized mounds of the mixture onto the prepared baking sheet.

- Bake for 18-20 minutes, or until the macaroons are golden brown.

- Allow to cool on the baking sheet before transferring to a wire rack to cool completely.

Baked Apples with Cinnamon

Description: These baked apples are sweetened with a touch of honey and spiced with cinnamon, creating a warm and comforting dessert that's both simple and healthy.

Prep Time: 10 minutes
Cook Time: 30 minutes
Serving: 4 servings

Nutritional Information: Calories: 120, Protein: 1g, Carbohydrates: 30g, Fat: 0g, Fiber: 5g

Ingredients:

- 4 medium apples, cored
- 1/4 cup raisins or chopped nuts (optional)
- 2 tablespoons honey
- 1 teaspoon ground cinnamon
- 1/4 cup water

Preparation Instructions:

- Preheat the oven to 350°F (175°C). Place the apples in a baking dish.
- Stuff each apple with raisins or nuts, if using.
- Drizzle honey over the apples and sprinkle with cinnamon.
- Pour water into the baking dish around the apples.

- Bake for 30 minutes, or until the apples are tender.
- Serve warm, optionally with a dollop of Greek yogurt.

Dark Chocolate Avocado Mousse

Description: This rich and creamy chocolate mousse uses avocado for a velvety texture and healthy fats. It's a decadent and nutritious dessert that's quick to prepare.

Prep Time: 10 minutes
Cook Time: 0 minutes
Serving: 4 servings

Nutritional Information: Calories: 220, Protein: 3g, Carbohydrates: 20g, Fat: 15g, Fiber: 6g

Ingredients:

- 2 ripe avocados, peeled and pitted
- 1/4 cup cocoa powder
- 1/4 cup maple syrup or honey
- 1/4 cup almond milk
- 1 teaspoon vanilla extract
- A pinch of salt

Preparation Instructions:

- In a blender or food processor, combine avocados, cocoa powder, maple syrup, almond milk, vanilla extract, and salt.

- Blend until smooth and creamy.
- Spoon the mousse into serving dishes and refrigerate for at least 1 hour before serving.

These dessert recipes offer a variety of sweet and satisfying options while keeping in mind the nutritional needs and preferences associated with the MTHFR diet. Enjoy these delicious and wholesome treats!

CHAPTER FOUR: Weekly Meal Plans

4-Week Meal Plan for Beginners

Week 1:

Monday

Breakfast: Green Power Smoothie

Lunch: Quinoa and Roasted Vegetable Salad

Dinner: Lemon Garlic Chicken with Steamed Broccoli

Snack: Spicy Roasted Chickpeas

Tuesday

Breakfast: Almond Flour Chocolate Chip Cookies (with a side of fruit)

Lunch: Turkey and Avocado Lettuce Wraps

Dinner: Baked Salmon with Sweet Potato Wedges

Snack: Veggie-Stuffed Hummus Dip with Carrot Sticks

Wednesday

Breakfast: Berry Blast Smoothie

Lunch: Chickpea and Spinach Salad

Dinner: Stir-Fried Tofu with Mixed Vegetables

Snack: Guacamole with Veggie Chips

Thursday

Breakfast: Tropical Delight Smoothie
Lunch: Lentil Soup
Dinner: Stuffed Bell Peppers with Ground Turkey
Snack: Coconut Macaroons

Friday

Breakfast: Chocolate Avocado Smoothie
Lunch: Grilled Chicken Caesar Salad
Dinner: Zucchini Noodles with Pesto Sauce
Snack: Baked Apples with Cinnamon

Saturday

Breakfast: Scrambled Eggs with Spinach and Tomatoes

Lunch: Tuna Salad with Mixed Greens

Dinner: Teriyaki Beef Stir-Fry

Snack: Almond-Crusted Cheese Bites

Sunday

Breakfast: Smoothie Bowl with Fresh Fruit and Seeds

Lunch: Chicken and Vegetable Soup

Dinner: Roasted Herb Chicken with Quinoa

Snack: Berry Chia Seed Pudding

Week 2:

Monday

Breakfast: Berry Chia Seed Pudding

Lunch: Grilled Chicken Wrap with Avocado and Veggies

Dinner: Shrimp and Asparagus Stir-Fry

Snack: Spicy Roasted Chickpeas

Tuesday

Breakfast: Green Power Smoothie

Lunch: Mediterranean Quinoa Salad

Dinner: Baked Cod with Lemon and Dill

Snack: Veggie-Stuffed Hummus Dip with Cucumber Slices

Wednesday

Breakfast: Tropical Delight Smoothie

Lunch: Beef and Vegetable Soup

Dinner: Stuffed Zucchini Boats

Snack: Guacamole with Veggie Chips

Thursday

Breakfast: Almond Flour Chocolate Chip Cookies (with a side of fruit)

Lunch: Spinach and Feta Stuffed Chicken

Dinner: Cauliflower Rice Stir-Fry

Snack: Coconut Macaroons

Friday

Breakfast: Chocolate Avocado Smoothie

Lunch: Turkey and Spinach Salad

Dinner: Grilled Salmon with Roasted Brussels Sprouts

Snack: Baked Apples with Cinnamon

Saturday

Breakfast: Smoothie Bowl with Fresh Fruit and Seeds

Lunch: Chicken and Avocado Lettuce Wraps

Dinner: Vegetable and Tofu Curry

Snack: Almond-Crusted Cheese Bites

Sunday

Breakfast: Berry Blast Smoothie

Lunch: Lentil and Vegetable Salad

Dinner: Herb-Crusted Pork Tenderloin with Roasted Vegetables

Snack: Dark Chocolate Avocado Mousse

Week 3:

Monday

Breakfast: Green Power Smoothie

Lunch: Chickpea and Avocado Salad

Dinner: Baked Chicken with Garlic and Herbs

Snack: Spicy Roasted Chickpeas

Tuesday

Breakfast: Berry Blast Smoothie

Lunch: Greek Salad with Grilled Chicken

Dinner: Stuffed Bell Peppers with Black Beans and Corn

Snack: Guacamole with Veggie Chips

Wednesday

Breakfast: Tropical Delight Smoothie

Lunch: Quinoa and Black Bean Bowl

Dinner: Lemon Herb Shrimp Skewers

Snack: Coconut Macaroons

Thursday

Breakfast: Almond Flour Chocolate Chip Cookies (with a side of fruit)

Lunch: Turkey and Sweet Potato Hash

Dinner: Zucchini and Tomato Baked Casserole

Snack: Baked Apples with Cinnamon

Friday

Breakfast: Chocolate Avocado Smoothie
Lunch: Spinach and Chicken Salad
Dinner: Grilled Pork Chops with Steamed Green Beans
Snack: Berry Chia Seed Pudding

Saturday

Breakfast: Smoothie Bowl with Fresh Fruit and Seeds
Lunch: Tuna and Avocado Salad
Dinner: Teriyaki Chicken with Cauliflower Rice
Snack: Almond-Crusted Cheese Bites

Sunday

Breakfast: Berry Blast Smoothie

Lunch: Chicken and Vegetable Stir-Fry

Dinner: Roasted Herb Salmon with Sweet Potatoes

Snack: Dark Chocolate Avocado Mousse

Week 4:

Monday

Breakfast: Tropical Delight Smoothie

Lunch: Mediterranean Chickpea Salad

Dinner: Baked Chicken Thighs with Roasted Carrots

Snack: Spicy Roasted Chickpeas

Tuesday

Breakfast: Berry Blast Smoothie

Lunch: Lentil and Vegetable Soup

Dinner: Stuffed Portobello Mushrooms

Snack: Guacamole with Veggie Chips

Wednesday

Breakfast: Chocolate Avocado Smoothie

Lunch: Grilled Vegetable and Hummus Wrap

Dinner: Shrimp and Broccoli Stir-Fry

Snack: Coconut Macaroons

Thursday

Breakfast: Almond Flour Chocolate Chip Cookies (with a side of fruit)
Lunch: Turkey and Avocado Salad
Dinner: Herb-Roasted Chicken with Quinoa
Snack: Baked Apples with Cinnamon

Friday

Breakfast: Green Power Smoothie
Lunch: Chicken and Vegetable Salad
Dinner: Stuffed Bell Peppers with Ground Beef
Snack: Berry Chia Seed Pudding

Saturday

Breakfast: Smoothie Bowl with Fresh Fruit and Seeds

Lunch: Spinach and Chicken Wrap

Dinner: Grilled Salmon with Cauliflower Rice

Snack: Almond-Crusted Cheese Bites

Sunday

Breakfast: Berry Blast Smoothie

Lunch: Tuna Salad with Mixed Greens

Dinner: Roasted Vegetable and Tofu Bowl

Snack: Dark Chocolate Avocado Mousse

Shopping Lists for Each Week

Week 1:

Produce: Spinach, kale, bananas, mango, broccoli, cherry tomatoes, cucumber, red bell pepper, black olives, avocados, apples, carrots, sweet potatoes, bell peppers, mixed greens, lemon, garlic

Protein: Chicken breast, salmon, ground turkey, eggs, tofu

Pantry: Almond milk, chia seeds, honey, coconut oil, dark chocolate chips, quinoa, chickpeas, hummus, nuts, coconut flour, almond flour

Spices/Condiments: Smoked paprika, cumin, chili powder, cayenne pepper, olive oil, vinegar, salt, pepper

Week 2:

Produce: Strawberries, blueberries, raspberries, spinach, mixed berries, apples, bell peppers, pineapple, bananas, cucumbers, zucchinis

Protein: Chicken, turkey, cod, shrimp

Pantry: Almond milk, chia seeds, honey, coconut oil, dark chocolate chips, coconut flour, almond flour, lentils

Spices/Condiments: Garlic powder, paprika, soy sauce, lemon juice

Week 3:

Produce: Spinach, avocados, apples, cucumbers, bell peppers, zucchini, broccoli, carrots, cherry tomatoes

Protein: Chicken, beef, cod, shrimp

Pantry: Almond milk, chia seeds, honey, almond flour, coconut flour, dark chocolate chips, quinoa, black beans

Spices/Condiments: Garlic, lemon, soy sauce, vinegar

Week 4:

Produce: Pineapple, berries, bananas, avocados, apples, bell peppers, carrots, broccoli, zucchini, mixed greens

Protein: Chicken, turkey, shrimp, tuna
Pantry: Almond milk, chia seeds, honey, almond flour, coconut flour, dark chocolate chips, quinoa, chickpeas, lentils

Spices/Condiments: Olive oil, garlic, lemon juice, soy sauce, herbs (such as rosemary, thyme)

Tips for Long-Term Success

Maintaining a Balanced Diet

Achieving and sustaining a balanced diet is crucial for long-term health and success with the MTHFR diet. Here are some essential tips to help you stay on track:

Variety is Key: Incorporate a wide range of foods in your diet to ensure you're getting a full spectrum of nutrients. Include plenty of fruits, vegetables, lean proteins, and healthy fats.

Portion Control: Pay attention to portion sizes to avoid overeating. Use smaller plates or bowls to help manage portions and listen to your body's hunger cues.

Mindful Eating: Eat slowly and without distractions. This helps you enjoy your food more and recognize when you're full, reducing the likelihood of overeating.

Plan Your Meals: Plan your meals and snacks ahead of time to ensure you always have nutritious options available. This also helps in avoiding last-minute unhealthy choices.

Stay Hydrated: Drink plenty of water throughout the day. Hydration is essential for overall health and can help with satiety and digestion.

Balance Macronutrients: Aim for a balance of carbohydrates, proteins, and fats in your meals. This helps maintain energy levels and supports overall health.

Incorporate Superfoods: Include nutrient-dense superfoods such as leafy greens, nuts, seeds, and berries to boost your diet's nutritional value.

Adapting Recipes to Your Preferences

Customizing recipes to suit your taste preferences and dietary needs can make maintaining the MTHFR diet more enjoyable and sustainable:

Substitute Ingredients: If you have allergies or dislike certain ingredients, find suitable substitutes. For example, use coconut flour instead of wheat flour, or swap dairy milk with almond milk.

Adjust Spices and Flavors: Experiment with different herbs and spices to make dishes more flavorful. This can help keep your meals interesting and enjoyable.

Try Different Cooking Methods: Change up the cooking methods (grilling, baking, steaming) to bring variety to your meals and maintain interest in your diet.

Portion Sizes: Adjust portion sizes based on your activity level and hunger. This flexibility allows you to tailor the diet to your lifestyle and needs.

Incorporate Personal Favorites: Include your favorite healthy ingredients or dishes in your meal plans. This can make the diet more enjoyable and easier to stick with.

Modify Recipes for Convenience: Simplify recipes to fit your schedule.

Prepare larger batches and freeze portions for quick and easy meals during busy times.

Staying Motivated and Consistent

Maintaining motivation and consistency is key to long-term success. Here are some strategies to help you stay on track:

Set Realistic Goals: Set achievable, short-term goals to build confidence and track progress. Celebrate milestones to keep yourself motivated.

Track Your Progress: Keep a food journal or use a tracking app to monitor your meals, progress, and how you feel.

This helps you stay accountable and make necessary adjustments.

Find Support: Join a community or support group with similar dietary goals. Sharing experiences and challenges can provide encouragement and accountability.

Experiment with New Recipes: Regularly try new recipes to keep your diet exciting and to discover new favorites. This prevents boredom and maintains interest.

Stay Flexible: Understand that occasional deviations from the diet are normal. Use them as learning experiences and return to your plan without guilt.

Focus on the Benefits: Remind yourself of the health benefits and improvements you're experiencing as a result of following the diet. This positive reinforcement can boost your motivation.

Self-Care: Incorporate self-care practices such as relaxation techniques, exercise, and adequate sleep. Overall well-being supports your ability to maintain a healthy diet.

By following these tips, you can create a balanced and enjoyable approach to the MTHFR diet, making it easier to achieve and maintain long-term success.

CONCLUSION

Navigating the MTHFR diet can be a transformative journey towards improved health and well-being. By embracing the principles outlined in this cookbook, you're not only enhancing your diet but also empowering yourself with the knowledge to make informed choices. The recipes and meal plans provided are designed to be both delicious and supportive of your genetic needs, ensuring that you can enjoy nutritious, satisfying meals every day.

Remember that consistency and balance are key. As you continue on this path, allow yourself the flexibility to adapt and evolve your diet according to your personal preferences and health goals. With commitment and creativity, the MTHFR diet can become a seamless and enjoyable part of your lifestyle.

Thank you for choosing this cookbook as your guide. Wishing you health, happiness, and a journey filled with vibrant, nourishing meals!

Acknowledgments

I would like to extend my heartfelt thanks to everyone who supported and contributed to the creation of this cookbook. Your encouragement, feedback, and support have been invaluable throughout this process.

Special thanks to:

My family and friends, whose patience and enthusiasm for taste-testing recipes kept me motivated.

Nutrition experts and health practitioners, for their insights and guidance on the MTHFR diet and its benefits.

The creative team behind the book, including editors, designers, who brought this vision to life.

Your support has made this project possible, and I am deeply grateful for each one of you.

About the Author

As an independent publisher and passionate advocate for health and wellness, I have dedicated my career to creating resources that empower individuals to take control of their health. With a background in nutrition and a love for cooking, I've crafted this cookbook to be both informative and enjoyable, helping you navigate the complexities of the MTHFR diet with ease and confidence. Thank you for joining me on this journey.